# Stress

## *The Psychology of Managing Pressure*

## *Practical Strategies to turn Pressure into Positive Energy*

## *(5 Key Stress Techniques for Stress, Anxiety, and Depression Relief)*

# PS: I Owe You!

Thank you for stopping by.

My name is Antony and I am passionate about teaching people literally everything I know about different aspects of life. I am an author and a ghostwriter. I run a small ghostwriting company with slightly over 100 writers. My wife (Faith) and I manage the business along with several other members of the team (editors).

Nice to meet you!

I started publishing (at Fantonpublishers.com) because I'd love to impart the knowledge I gather every single day in my line of work (reading and editing over 10 ghostwritten books every single day). My ghostwriting company deals with literally every topic under the sun, which puts me at a very unique position to learn more in a month than I learnt in my 4 years as a Bachelor of Commerce, Accounting, student. I am constantly answering questions from my friends, relatives and even strangers on various topics that I come across every day at work.

After several years of helping people to achieve different goals (e.g. weight loss, making money online, human resources, management, investing, stress reduction, depression, budgeting, saving etc.) offline thanks to my 'street' as well as 'class' knowledge on different topics, I realized I could be of better help to the world by publishing what I learn. My books are a reflection of what I have been gathering over the years. That's why they are not just focused on one niche but every niche possible out there.

If you would love to be part of my lovely audience who want to change multiple aspects of their life, subscribe to our newsletter http://bit.ly/2fantonpubnewbooks or follow us on social media to receive notifications whenever we publish new books on any niche. You can also send me an email; I would love to hear from you!

**PS**: Valuable content is my bread and butter. And since I have lots of it to go around, I can share it freely (not everything is about money - **changing lives comes first!**)

*I promise; I am busy just as you are and won't spam (I hate spam too)!*

**Antony,**

**Website**: http://www.fantonpublishers.com/

**Email:** Support@fantonpublishers.com

**Twitter**: https://twitter.com/FantonPublisher

**Facebook Page**:
https://www.facebook.com/Fantonpublisher/

**Private Facebook Group For Readers:**
https://www.facebook.com/groups/FantonPublishers/

**Pinterest**: https://www.pinterest.com/fantonpublisher/

### *Some of the best things in life are free, right?*

As a sign of good faith, I will start by giving out content that will help you to implement not only everything I teach in this book but in every other book I write. The content is about life transformation, presented in bit size pieces for easy implementation. I believe that without such a checklist, you are likely to have a hard time implementing anything in this book and any other thing you set out to do religiously and sticking to it for the long haul. It doesn't matter whether your goals relate to weight loss, relationships, personal finance, investing, personal development, improving communication in your family, your overall health, finances, improving your sex life, resolving issues in your relationship, fighting PMS successfully, investing, running a successful business, traveling etc. With a checklist like the one I will show you, you can bet that anything you do will seem a lot easier to implement until the end. This checklist will help you to start well and not lose steam along the way, until the very end.

Therefore, even if you don't continue reading this book, at least read the one thing that will help you in every other aspect of your life.

Send me a message on support@fantonpublishers.com and I will send you my 5 Pillar Life Transformation Checklist.

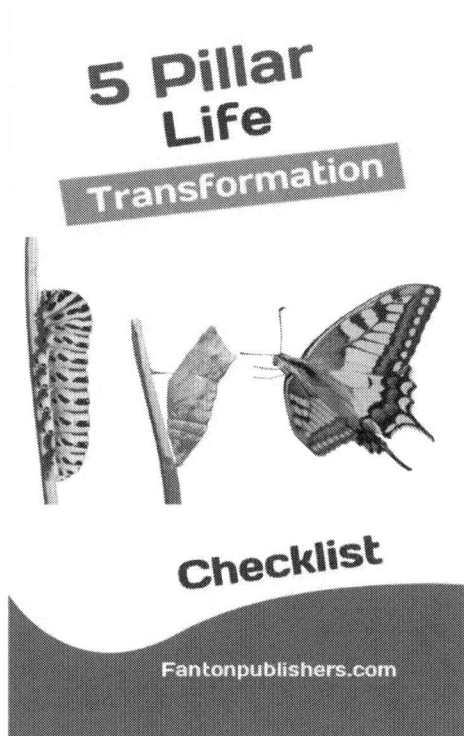

*Your life will never be the same again (if you implement what's in this book), I promise.*

*Your life will never be the same again (if you implement what's in this book), I promise.*

# Introduction

Stress and its attendant psychological disorders such as depression and anxiety are some of the major causes of ailments and low productivity among the active workforce. More worrisome is the fact that despite the number of research studies conducted annually to find a lasting solution to this problem, it is still a menace in today's society.

The number of stressors we face continues to increase everyday thanks to the highly demanding nature of today's jobs and businesses. From meeting your daily targets in the workplace to running the home, several things that relate to our modern day life can scuttle your peace of mind and affect your overall mood and outlook to life. These stressors never seem to stop coming.

If you are the empathic type with an empathic nature, you even face far more stressors than the average person does because you will react emotionally to things happening around the world and to news concerning anyone you know in the same way you would react if they were issues that affect you personally.

And the sad thing is that there seems to be a direct link between stress, anxiety, and depression as all three or at least two can occur concurrently. It is easy to get into a depressed state when you feel stressed, or once depressed, be anxious.

Whichever one applies to you, this book is designed to address these three major mental conditions, help you understand what you are dealing with, and provide you with 5 key techniques that can help you overcome these problems.

Let's begin.

# Table of Contents

Before we start discussing the different strategies that you can use to fight stress, anxiety and depression, it is important that you start by having an understanding of the link between the 3 mental health issues so you know what you are up against. As they say, knowing your enemy is the first step to winning any war.

## Understanding the Biological Link between Stress, Anxiety & Depression

Let us understand the link between stress, anxiety, and depression before we go into techniques to beat this trio.

Researchers from the University of Ontario, Canada have this to say about the biological link between these three conditions, why one can bring about the other, and why the same techniques are effective against the three. According to Stephen Ferguson, a lead researcher at the aforementioned University, the connecting mechanism found in the human brain explains how being stressed up and anxious can make you depressed.

According to the results of the findings published online in the *Nature Neuroscience* journal, findings from this research suggest that the same drugs and treatment techniques could be selectively used to treat depressive disorders that could result from past stressful experiences.

As discovered in the research, the linking mechanism in the brain shows the interaction between the corticotrophin releasing factor receptor and certain types of serotonin receptors. The study further proved that the corticotrophin releasing factor receptor works to increase the number of serotonin receptors on cell surfaces in the human brain. This increase can lead to a level of abnormal signaling.

Since the corticotrophin receptors lead to anxiety in response to stress, and the serotonin receptors lead to depression, the research clearly shows how stress, anxiety, and depression pathways connect through very distinct processes in the human brain.

While most major depressive disorders often occur concurrently with anxiety disorders in most people, the causes for both the depression and the anxiety strongly links to very stressful experiences. In addition, there is scientific proof that stressful experiences can make the symptoms of depression and anxiety severe.

Identifying the link between these three has made it easy to choose the best treatment techniques to deal with stress and the other disorders that go along with it.

Having seen the connection between stress and its accomplices i.e. depression and anxiety, let us now see how stress affects different areas of your life.

# How Stress Affects You

If there is one thing you should pay urgent attention to, it is your stress levels and the major stressors you have to deal with. Stress affects your life more than you have ever thought possible. The fact that you are not aware of the level of damage stress inflicts on you does not mean its negative effects are not as widespread as they are debilitating.

Apart from the anxiety and depressive disorders that accompany most cases of high stress levels, stress also affects your life in a number of negative ways. Below are some common ways stress affects different areas of your life and why you should deal with high stress levels as soon as possible:

## Cognitive Effects of Stress

1.  **Poor judgment:** High stress level has a way of clouding your sense of judgment primarily because of your inability to reason out issues objectively and intelligently.

2.  **Memory problems:** People with cases of high stress levels and its attendant mental disorders also battle issues related to memory loss and inability to remember things in details.

3.  **Brain fog:** One common symptom of stress most people experience is mental fatigue or confusion. This will also happen when you are either anxious or depressed. Its main characteristics are irrational thoughts running

15

through your mind at the same time, which leaves you fuzzy and disoriented.

4. **Lack of concentration:** It is impossible to concentrate on anything when your stress levels are at an all-time high. This is why people with high stress levels often lack motivation and the will power to get anything done.

5. **Indecision:** When you cannot concentrate because of high stress levels, it becomes increasingly difficult to make important decisions, which is why a high stress level often causes very low productivity in all areas of your life.

6. **Self-doubt:** High stress level, anxiety, and depression have a way of making you think you are not worth your salt. When you cannot seem to find your bearing, it is easy to feel inferior to others around you, which can easily lead to loss of direction.

7. **Starting several tasks and achieving very little:** In his confusion, a highly stressed person might try to get busy at several things at the same time. This is because of the confused state of mind that comes with stress. The result is dismal achievement at the end of the day.

## Emotional Effects of Stress

1. **Depression:** Of course, this one goes hand-in-hand with stress—as we have reiterated severally. Once your stress level stays high and unchecked for long, depression

follows suit because of your inability to focus and concentrate on anything.

2. **Irritability:** Feeling easily irritated is a common adverse effect of stress. High stress levels will make you feel irritated at almost everything and everyone. This is why you see stressed people showing unexplainable anger and snapping at others at the slightest provocation.

3. **Panic:** Your high stress level will make you anxious and fearful when you have no reason to be. This is why panic disorders seem to accompany almost every case of chronic stress. Stress will keep your heart racing and skipping beats at the slightest scare.

4. **Moodiness:** A highly stressed person can be the moodiest person you can ever find anywhere. Stress comes with low spirits, lack of enthusiasm, loss of motivation and the likes, which explains why you are most likely to feel moody and unexcited when stressed out.

5. **Frustration:** Stress will make you want to give up because of frustration. This explains why people with chronic stress fall into depression easily and think suicidal thoughts.

## Physical Effects of Stress

1. **Fatigues, Pains, and aches:** High stress levels will make you feel constant chest pains, aches, and fatigues.

This is most common when you wake every morning after having your sleep disrupted by panic attacks and incoherent nightmares.

2. **Skin problems:** Some people with high stress level have reported an outbreak of skin problems such as acne, rashes, eczema, etc. This links back to the fact that stress affects the production of certain hormones and chemicals in the body.

3. **Indigestion:** Digestive disorders are common symptoms of stress. Stress can cause you to experience constant constipation, indigestion, and other such stomach-related problems.

4. **Rapid Heartbeat:** Your accelerated heart rate is one of the ways your body tells you it is undergoing intense pressure and needs urgent help. When such high stress levels remain unchecked for long, they can easily deteriorate into serious health problems such as high blood pressure.

## Behavioral Effects of Stress

1. **Increased use of alcohol, cigarettes, and caffeine:** Stress can cause you to resort to certain unhealthy habits as a way of escape. However, most of the habits picked up as a way of dealing with stress are negative habits that end up making your situation worse. Habits such as drinking too much alcohol, smoking cigarettes, getting

high on drugs and other intoxicating substances are common in people dealing with stress and depression.

2. **Lack of motivation:** Stress will take away your fighting spirit. It is hard to keep it together when stress is taking its toll on your mind and body. With a confused mind and a weak body, you can do very few things and therefore, the earlier you deal with your stress issues, the sooner you can get your life back on track.

3. **Sleep disorders:** Stress is a known notorious sleep thief. Inadequate sleep and stress often go hand-in-hand. If you have been experiencing sleeplessness, it could be a good sign you need to pay more attention to dealing with stress.

4. **Living in isolation:** Stress will make you recline into your shell in an attempt to stay away from others who seem to be having the best time of their lives. Isolation only makes the condition worse. Hanging out with positive and fun people will do you much good.

Let us see how the stress response work and how activating the relaxation response with the right relaxation techniques can counter it and help you relax:

# How the Stress Response Works

Specifically, we are going to look at the role of relaxation techniques for activating the relaxation response to counteract the natural stress response.

## Relaxation Techniques

Many people assume relaxing in front of the TV is enough to make them de-stress at the end of a very stressful day. The truth remains that when it comes to beating stress, there is more to relaxation than chilling out in front of your TV set chewing your favorite popcorn.

When it comes to beating stress, you need relaxation techniques that can help you activate the relaxation response.

### Relaxation Response

Whenever your stress levels get so high that your nervous system becomes overwhelmed, your body gets a boosted supply of "fight or flight" hormones. This stress response can be a real lifesaver during life-threatening emergencies where there is need for you to act very quickly. However, when the stresses of your day-to-day life and challenges constantly activate this response, it can wear you down both physically and emotionally.

While it may not be possible to avoid stress entirely, it is possible to counteract the very detrimental effects of stress by learning how to produce this all-important relaxation response, a state of deep rest considered to be the exact opposite of the stress response. This relaxation response helps bring your mind and body into the natural state of equilibrium.

Some of the things that happen when your relaxation response activates are:

1. Your muscle relax

2. Your blood pressure drops

3. Your heart rate normalizes

4. Your breathing slows down

5. Your blood flow to the brain increases.

Here, we will discuss the ability of key relaxation techniques to bring about this relaxation response; that these techniques bring about the relaxation response is what makes them ideal for fighting stress, depression, anxiety, fear and tension.

Below are the 5 key relaxation techniques you can engage in to get instant relief from stress and other mental disorders beginning with yoga:

# 1st Technique: Yoga Poses for Relaxation and Calmness

Yoga has the ability to combat both stress and tension effectively. In addition, regular practice, yoga will help increase your resilience when those recurring stress triggers rear up their ugly heads.

While any type of yoga is generally a good way to combat stress, we have a number of specific poses that have proven to have awesome stress-beating effects. Below are the most potent of these yoga asanas (poses):

## The Eagle Pose (Garudasana)

This yoga pose requires that you focus your mind on a single point, which is why it is a very powerful stress and tension management tool. It is also ideal for freeing up tightness around the hips and shoulders—common accumulation points for emotional stress.

### *Steps to the eagle pose:*

1. Assume the tadasana pose (shown below), and from there, keep your feet hip-width apart while keeping your arms as widely spread as possible. Bring your right arm over your left arm.

2. Then, bend your elbows and bring your palms together.

3. Shift your weight to the four corners of your right foot and bend your knees a little bit.

4.  Lift your left thigh up and place it over your right thigh. If your knees feel comfortable and you are able to hook your toes behind your right calf, do so. You can leave the foot where it is if you cannot do the toe-hooking stunt. You do not have to force it: it's an anatomical feat some people can pull off naturally.

5.  Engage your core and start sinking your hips down while you maintain the length of your spine. Firmly keep your gaze on the point you chose to focus on as your breath flows effortlessly.

6.  To come out of this pose, begin to unwind slowly until you have returned to the Tadasana pose. You can repeat the pose on your other side.

**TIP:** The object you choose to fix your gaze on is an important part of the stress-relieving pose. As such, make sure you choose to focus on something that lifts your spirit naturally such as a gemstone or crystal.

# The Standing Forward Fold (Uttanasana)

The Uttanasana pose can help you achieve a quiet and calm mind, balance your nervous system, and promote feelings of peace. It also energetically balances your <u>sacral chakra,</u> which when overstimulated, can contribute to excessive and fluctuating emotional energy. Uttanasana can help quiet a busy mind, balance the nervous system, and promote feelings of calm and peace.

## *Steps to the Uttanasana pose:*

1. Start with the Tadasana pose, bend your knees, engage your core slightly, hinge forward from your hips, and then place your hands either in front of you or alongside your feet.

2.  Shift your weight to the balls of your feet and feel your sit bones lifting upwards. For very tight hamstrings, you can keep your knees bent to keep your lower back protected. Alternatively, you can lengthen through the backs of your legs as you keep your weight on the balls of your feet.

3.  Take hold of each one of your elbows with your opposite hand and soften around your neck, eyes, jaw, neck, head, and mind.

4.  You can hold this pose for as long as you feel comfortable. Take your time coming out of this pose if you have any history of low blood pressure.

**TIP:** To enhance the stress and anxiety-relieving effect of this pose, visualize your worries melting away from the top of your head and absorbed by the ground around you literarily.

# Child's Pose (Balasana)

Whenever you feel frazzled, you tend to put lots of pressure on your adrenal glands, which can always lead to burnout and increased stress. The child pose is quite soothing for adrenals and therefore, doing the child pose often can give you the effect of a bubble bath, giant hug, and a bowl of soup all in one package.

## *Steps to the Balasana pose:*

1.  Stay down on your hands and knees, and then take the sit-bones back over your heels and your hands out in front of you. Fold your torso forward in a very slow move until you can feel your eyebrow touching the center of your yoga mat.

2.  You can keep your knees together or separate them a bit wider than your hips; whichever way, make sure your toes are touching.

3.  Keep your arms traditionally resting back alongside your body with your palms held up, but make sure you can

stack your forearms and hands and still rest your head there if you think that is more preferable.

4. If your butt or hips are not touching your heels, you can simply place a cushion in between to help you let go and relax more. Hold the pose for 10 breaths or more and let go as much as possible with each exhalation.

5. Visualize a soothing color at the eyebrow center such as lilac, gold, or blue. Imagine that color flowing in and out of each breath you take, calming and soothing your mind as you go.

# The Thunderbolt Pose (Vajrasana)

The thunderbolt has a powerful soothing effect on your mind and body. If your high stress levels and tension give you digestive problems, this pose will help you relieve it.

## *Steps to the Thunderbolt pose:*

1. Get on your knees, and from the kneeling position, sit back on your heels. You can keep a cushion between your sit-bones and your feet if you feel comfortable enough with that.

2. Maintain a straight spine, and feel your crown draw up towards the ceiling.

3. Cross your hands in front of your chest and cup your palms at your underarms. Keep your thumps up in front of you.

4. Connect with your breath as you notice how fast your mind starts calming and slowing down. Hold the pose for about 10 minutes and imagine yourself releasing stress and tension with every breath you exhale.

5. If you are not comfortable sitting on your knees for that long, you can cross your legs.

**TIP:** Do this before bedtime every night to help you enjoy better sleep at night.

# Reclined Bound Angle Pose (Supta Baddha Konasana)

This pose will make you feel like you have embarked on a mini stress-relieving vacation. It can help you open through the inner thighs, hips, and groin; all of the places where you can hold stress and tension. The floor beneath you will give you the support you need to surrender to the moment and practice the calming art of letting go.

## *Steps to the Reclined Bound Angle pose:*

1. Lie on your back in a <u>Savasana pose</u>. Bring the soles of your feet together, with your knees out to the side. If one or both of your knees are a bit far from the floor, you can use yoga blocks, folded blankets, or bolsters underneath them in order to ensure the pose is more soothing.

2. As for your arms, you can lift them overhead and take each one of your elbows with your opposite hands, or you can keep them resting on the floor alongside your torso. Alternatively, you can place one hand on your belly and

31

the other on your heart center to create a soothing connection within you.

3. Stay for as long as you feel comfortable and move slowly when you are finally ready to come out of this pose.

**TIP:** This gives you a great opportunity to reinforce a very positive and calming message to yourself. You can add a mantra or positive affirmation to every inhalation and exhalation such as "I choose to be relaxed and calm" as you inhale and "I let go of all stress, worries and anxieties" as you exhale.

# The Corpse Pose (Savasana)

This is the easiest yoga pose to do physically, but many yogis consider it the most difficult for the mind to master.

## ***Steps to the Corpse pose:***

1. Lie still on your yoga mat, with your arms placed on both sides, palms facing upwards, legs relaxed, and your feet turning towards the side of your mat.

2. If you feel tension at your lower back, you can support it with a pillow.

3. Slowly close the eyes and consciously release any tension in your face

4. Practice deep breathing until you are very relaxed. Stay in the moment and refuse to dwell on any invading thoughts

We mentioned deep breathing casually in some of the yoga poses. Let us now see what deep breathing is all about and how you can harness its benefits as one of the key techniques for combating stress and its attendant problems in your day-to-day life.

# 2nd Technique: Deep breathing For Stress and Anxiety Relief

When done accurately, deep breathing can bring instant relief to your stress, anxiety, and depression thanks to its very calming effects.

Let us begin by learning how to breathe properly:

## How to Breath (Deep Breathe) Properly

As strange as it may sound, most people do not know how to breathe properly. Natural breathing should involve the whole of your diaphragm and a large muscle in your abdomen.

Your belly should expand whenever you breathe in and fall as you breathe out. We call this diaphragmatic breathing. People forget the right way to breathe overtime, which is the major cause of the stress and anxiety because it causes shallow breaths that we take with using our shoulders and chest alone.

Well, even if you have been doing the breathing thing the wrong way for so long, it is never too late to unlearn the wrong breathing pattern in order to relearn the right pattern as a way of keeping yourself protected from stress.

Here are some simple steps you can take to improve your breathing:

1. Find a very comfortable position such as sitting or lying on your back. If you choose to sit, make sure your back is

straight and the tensions on your shoulders released by allowing the shoulders to drop.

2. Close your eyes so that you can focus on the mechanics of breathing rather than focus on outside stimuli.

3. Place one of your hands on your chest and the other on your stomach

4. Take in a few deep breaths. Take note of how your belly rises with each inhalation and falls with each exhalation.

5. Keep practicing deep breathing until you can associate in breaths and out breaths with the rising and falling of your belly.

## Basic Deep Breathing Tips You Will Find Useful

1. Relearning how to breathe can take some time. However, this art will become easier with frequent practices. You can take out some time every day to engage in deep breathing exercises. The good thing about practicing deep breathing to beat stress is that you can do it almost anywhere and at any time of the day.

2. Try practicing whenever you feel calm and relaxed. This will make taking in deep breaths easier for you.

3. If you find it hard to take in deep breaths, try breathing in through your nostrils and exhaling through your mouth.

You can also count to 5 mentally whenever you breathe in and out.

4. With time, you can tell how long you practice before you feel relieved from stress, tension, or anxiety. You can set time limits as a beginner, like, 3 minutes per session, several times a day. Always remember that it is more beneficial to practice several short breaths a day than to engage in a single long deep breathing episode. Practicing more often will help incorporate deep breathing into your daily life and schedules.

Let us now talk about the progressive muscle relaxation technique:

# 3ʳᵈ Technique: Progressive Muscle Relaxation Anxiety, Depression, Stress & Tension Relief

This is a two-step process where you systematically tense and relax different group of muscles in your body. If practiced regularly, you become intimately familiar with that muscle tension that tells you your body needs rest. This familiarity will teach you to react swiftly and accordingly to the very first signs of muscular tension that accompany stress.

Your body's relaxation goes hand-in-hand with your mind relaxation—just in case you start wondering how relaxing your muscles helps you deal with anxiety and depression. For enhanced results, you can combine progressive muscle relaxation with other relaxation techniques such as deep breathing.

## How to Practice Progressive Muscle Relaxation

If you have ever had any issues of back problems, muscle spasms, or other such serious injuries that may have led to tension in your muscles, you may need to consult your doctor before you embark on this muscle relaxation technique.

### *Here is what to do:*

1. The idea is to begin at your feet and work your way up to your facial muscles (or the other way round).

2. Loosen your clothes, take your shoes off, and get as comfortable as possible.

3. Take a couple of minutes to practice deep breathing

4. When you are set, simply shift all attention to your right foot. Take some minutes to understand how the foot feels at that moment.

5. Slowly tense the muscles of the right foot, squeezing those muscles as tightly as possible. You can hold and count from 1-10.

6. Relax your foot before focusing on the tension as it flows away from your right foot and note how the foot feels as it becomes loose and limp.

7. Stay in this state of relaxation briefly and breathe in slowly, but deeply.

8. Shift all attention to your left foot and follow the same process you used for the right foot.

9. Slowly move up through the body, where you contract as well as relax the various muscle groups while going up.

10. This will take some regular practices at first, but always make sure you never tense any other muscles save the ones you are focusing on at any point

Here is a good muscle relaxation sequence you can work with:

1. Right foot

2. Left foot

3. Right calf

4. Left calf

5. Hips and buttocks

6. Stomach

7. Chest

8. Back

9. Right arm and hand

10. Left arm and hand

11. Neck and shoulders

12. Face

# 4ᵗʰ Technique: Body Scan Meditation for Stress and Anxiety Relief

The body scan meditation is a form of meditation that focuses your whole attention on different parts of the body. Just like the progressive muscle relaxation technique that we discussed earlier, you begin with the feet and then work all the way up to your facial muscles.

It differs from the progressive muscle relaxation in that in this instance, you do not need to tense your muscles. You simply focus on how each part feels, without judging the feeling as either positive or negative.

## How to Practice Body Scan Meditation

Here are steps to the muscle scan meditation:

1. Lie on your back and keep your arms relaxed at your sides without crossing your legs. You can leave your eyes open or closed.

2. Focus on your right toes. Take note of any sensation present in those toes even as you focus on your breathing. Imagine each of the deep breaths you take flowing to your toes. Maintain your focus on that area for 1-3 minutes.

3. Move that focus to the right sole. Become aware of the sensation on your right sole and imagine each breath you take flowing from the right sole. Maintain your focus for 1-3 minutes before moving it to your right ankle.

4. Move your focus to your calf, then the knee, followed by thigh, and then the hip and repeat the sequence for your left leg beginning with the toes and ending with the left hipbone. From there, you can then move to your torso, through your lower back abdomen, your upper back, your chest, and your shoulders. If you get to any part that gives you some pain and discomfort, pay closer attention and spend longer there until you sense the tension and pain drifting away.

5. Once done with your body scan, relax for some minutes—say 5-7 minutes—in stillness and silence, taking note of how your body feels. You can then slowly open your eyes and stretch if need be.

Now comes the chief of all relaxation techniques: the mindfulness meditation technique. Each one of the techniques we have mentioned thus far draws strength from this one.

# 5th Technique: Mindfulness Meditation

Mindfulness meditation is a relaxation technique that can help you switch your focus from past regrets and future worries to what is happening around you at any given moment. This allows you to engage fully in the present moment and helps you enjoy life as it happens, which is why it is highly effective for combating stress, anxiety and depression.

For ages, man has used meditations that cultivate mindfulness to reduce stress, anxiety, depression, and all other negative mood disorders. Some mindful meditation techniques help you focus on one single repetitive action such as deep breathing, a few mantras, positive self-talks/affirmations, or the flickering light of a candle.

The good thing about mindful meditation is that once it becomes a part of your daily life, you can easily translate mindfulness into your normal daily routines and do things with increased concentration and accuracy. Other activities you can do mindfully to further win the battle with stress, anxiety, and depression include mindful walking, dancing, workout, eating, bath, washing, home chores, etc.

## Basic Mindfulness Meditation

Here are the basic steps to mindful meditation:

1.  Get yourself comfortably seated on a straight-back chair or sit cross-legged on the floor.

2. Choose one aspect of your breathing and focus on it such as the sound of air rushing in and out of your airways, the sensation of inhalation and exhalation, the rise and fall of your belly, etc.

3. The moment your concentration narrows, start widening your focus and become aware of every sound, thought, and sensation present.

4. Embrace and consider every sensation or thought without being judgmental. If you catch your thoughts straying at any point, simply bring it back to focus on that aspect of your breathing you chose before widening your awareness once more.

You can get more from your mindful meditation sessions by incorporating two powerful relaxation tools: visualization and positive self-talks:

# 1: Visualization

You can incorporate visualization into your mindful meditation sessions. However, it can be a powerful tool for the treatment of stress, depression, and anxiety on its own.

Visualization, also called guided imagery, involves imagining a scene that makes you feel at peace and free from every trace of anxiety and tension. Choose whatever you find most appealing and peaceful such as your favorite childhood spot, a quiet forest path, a tropical beach, a riverbank, an ocean view, etc.

You can practice visualization with the aid of listening aids such as soothing music, recordings that match your chosen setting, sound machine, or in silence. If you have chosen to visualize a beach, the sound of ocean waves will be ideal.

### *Steps to visualization:*

1. Close your eyes and imagine a peaceful setting.

2. Picture the setting as vividly as possible: see, hear, smell, taste, and feel everything in that setting. Visualization works best when all sensory details involving all the senses are incorporated. If you are imagining a dock for instance, see the sun set over the water, hear the birds sing, smell the pine trees, feel the coldness of the water as it overflows the riverbank and touches your bare feet, taste the clean, and fresh air.

3. Imagine your worries, anxieties, and fears drifting away as you explore your serene environment and enjoy its restfulness.

4. When done, calmly open your eyes and return to the present. You will be amazed at how calm and relaxed you will feel.

## 2: Positive Self-Talk

If your 5-year old son were to tell you he is nervous about going to school the next day, what would be your response? You are not likely to tell the child he is being dumb and behaving like a sissy. You would probably want to find out if the child is a victim of is bullying or why he feels nervous about going to school.

We seem so good at helping people we care about deal with stress and stressors in their lives, and yet find it difficult to handle our own stress issues.

In the same way you would reassure your child there is nothing to be anxious about, you should learn to use some positive self-talks on yourself whenever you feel nervous, stressed out, or tensed up.

Here are some examples of phrases you can coin into positive self-talks and incorporate into your mindful meditation session to help you feel more comfortable and relaxed when there are reasons for nerves to become ruffled:

1. "I have been through worse issues in the past; I will get through this as well."

2. "This feeling shall pass."

3. "There is no reason to panic or feel anxious right now."

4. "All is well with me and all that are mine."

5. "I feel safe right now."

6. "I have the power to make myself calm despite the anxiety I feel right now."

7. "I can feel my taut muscles relaxing and my heart rate slowing down."

**NOTE:** These meditations become more successful when done in very serene and private environments where the chances of interruption are minimal. Also, make sure you experiment with different sitting positions to know one you are most comfortable with. Avoid lying down as it may make you sleep off during meditation.

# Final Tips to Help You Live a Stress-Free Life

The following tips build on what we have learnt thus far:

## Know your stressors and avoid them

You should be able to identify what triggers your stress and avoid such triggers. Know friends whose company makes you feel terrible about life and stay away from them. Know places you visit and come home in very low spirits and avoid such places. Know habits that make you sick and negative such as gluttony, drunkenness, late night movies, social media addictions and avoid them.

## Embrace minimalism

Learn to be satisfied with little. Reduce your number of friends, your daily tasks, and activities, de-clutter your home, get rid of useless clutter, and keep only things you really need. This will reduce your workload, increase the amount of free time with which you get practice the 5 key techniques discussed in this guide, and give you more peace of mind with increased productivity.

## Pay attention to your diet

It may surprise you to know that what you eat and drink most times affect your mood more than you would have ever thought possible. Foods containing alcohol and caffeine often associate with worsened cases of anxiety disorders.

According to studies, even the slightest amount of caffeine can cause panic attacks, bouts of anxiety, increased nervousness, and irritability when consumed.

## Get adequate sleep

Almost all of us feel a bit crabby after what we can only call a rough night's sleep. Most people dealing with emotional disorders have disrupted sleep to wrestle with every night. Sometimes it is not easy to tell which one started before the other between the high stress levels and poor sleep habits. According to a study conducted by researchers at Pennsylvania University, losing a few hours of sleep can increase your stress, exhaustion, anger, and sadness levels.

## Stay Fit and active

We all know how important daily physical exercises are to our body and overall health. Research studies conducted in the last couple of decades suggest that exercise is far more effective than medications.

Maintaining a healthy exercise routine minimizes stress, enhance self-esteem, increase your energy levels, and enhance your mood. During these physical exercises, your body releases chemicals known as endorphins, chemicals that can interact with receptors in your brain to cause those feelings of euphoria and conceal physical pains.

## Build better connections

You need to make new friends who can bring new excitement and sunshine into your life. The more fun you have, the less time you will have to worry about a future you cannot influence and regret past mistakes you cannot correct. Stay away from toxic people and learn to say no to people and activities that eat up your productive time and keep you disorganized.

## Engage yourself meaningfully

Find a new cause or hobby that will challenge, excite, and keep you occupied. You can volunteer for a nonprofit and engage in more outdoor campaigns to let in some more sunshine into your life and bring in some positive value to the world you live in.

# Conclusion

We have come to the end of the book. Thank you for reading and congratulations for reading until the end.

It may not be entirely possible to live without stress, anxiety or depression as no one can accurately predict tomorrow. However, with the techniques and tips outlined in this book, you can manage your stress effectively and keep them as low as possible at all times.

If you found the book valuable, can you recommend it to others? One way to do that is to post a review on Amazon.

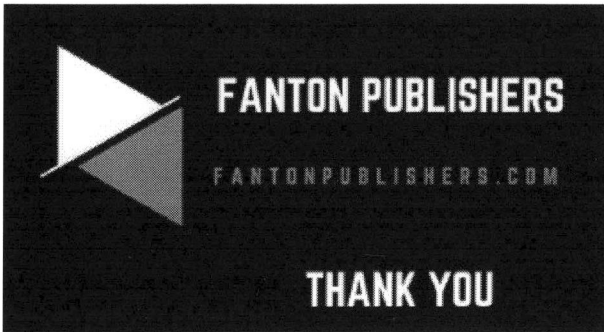

**FANTON PUBLISHERS**

FANTONPUBLISHERS.COM

**THANK YOU**

# Do You Like My Book & Approach To Publishing?

If you like my writing and style and would love the ease of learning literally everything you can get your hands on from Fantonpublishers.com, I'd really need you to do me either of the following favors.

# 6 Things

I'll be honest; publishing books on what I learn in my line of work gives me satisfaction. But the biggest satisfaction that I can get as an author is knowing that I am influencing people's lives positively through the content I publish. Greater joy even comes from knowing that customers appreciate the great content that they have read in every book through giving feedback, subscribing to my newsletter, sending emails to tell me how transformative the content they read is, following me on social media and buying several of my books. That's why I am always seeking to engage my readers at a personal level to know them and for them to know me, not just as an author but as a person because we all want to belong. That's why I strive to use different channels to engage my readers so that I can ultimately build a cordial relationship with them for our mutual success i.e. I succeed as an author while at the same time my readers learn stuff that takes days and sometimes weeks to write, edit, format and publish in a matter of hours.

To build this relationship, I'd really appreciate if you could do any or all the following:

## 1: First, I'd Love It If You Leave a Review of This Book on Amazon.

Let me be honest; reviews play a monumental role in determining whether customers purchase different products online. From the thousands of other books that are on Amazon about the topic, you chose to read this one. I am grateful for that. I may not know why you read my book, especially until the end considering the fact that most readers don't read until the end. Perhaps you purchased this book after reading some of the reviews and were glued with reading the book because it was educative and engaging. Even if you didn't read it because of the positive reviews, perhaps you can make the next customer's purchasing decision a lot easier by posting a review of this book on Amazon!

I'd love it if you did that, as this would help me spread word out about my books and publishing business. The more the readers, the bigger a community we build and we all benefit! If you could leave your honest review of this book on Amazon, I'd be forever grateful (well, I am already grateful to you for purchasing the book and reading it until the end- I don't' take that for granted!). Please Leave a Review of This Book on Amazon.

## 2: <u>Check Out My Other Books</u>

As I stated earlier, my biggest joy in all this is building an audience that loves my approach to publishing and the amazing content I publish. I know every author has his/her style. Mine is publishing what I learn to readers out there so that they can learn what is trending, what other readers are also searching for in the nonfiction world and much more. As such, if you <u>read the other books I have published</u>, you will undoubtedly know a lot more than the average person on a diverse range of issues. And as you well know, knowledge is power- and the biggest investment that you can ever have on your life!

**PS:** If you want me to filter everything for you to include only Ketogenic diet books, you can <u>subscribe to my newsletter</u> and I will send you a list of all my Ketogenic diet books along with other useful content that I come across to ensure you succeed while at it <u>http://bit.ly/2Cketodietfanton</u>.

## 3: Let's Get In Touch

Let's get closer than just leaving reviews and buying my other books. Reach out to me through email, like or follow me on social media and let's interact. You will perhaps get to know stuff about me that will change your life in a way. As we interact, we will also influence each other in a way. I' definitely would love to learn something from you as we get to know each other.

**Antony**

**Website**: http://www.fantonpublishers.com/

**Email:** Support@fantonpublishers.com

**Twitter**: https://twitter.com/FantonPublisher

**Facebook** **Page**: https://www.facebook.com/Fantonpublisher/

**My Ketogenic Diet Books Page:** **https://www.facebook.com/pg/Fast-Keto-Meals-336338180266944**

**Private Facebook Group For Readers:** https://www.facebook.com/groups/FantonPublishers/

**Pinterest**: https://www.pinterest.com/fantonpublisher/

## 4: Grab Some Freebies On Your Way Out; Giving Is Receiving, Right?

I gave you 2 freebies at the start of the book, one on general life transformation and one about the Ketogenic diet. You are free to choose either or both!

**Ketogenic Diet Freebie**: http://bit.ly/2fantonpubketo

**5 Pillar Life Transformation Checklist**: http://bit.ly/2fantonfreebie

## 5: Suggest Topics That You'd Love Me To Cover To Increase Your Knowledge Bank. As I

stated, I love feedback; any type of feedback- positive or negative. As such, make sure to reach out. I am looking forward to seeing your suggestions and insights on the topic. You could even suggest improvements to this book. Simply send me a message on Support@fantonpublishers.com. As a publisher, I strive to publish content that my readers are actively looking for. Therefore, your input is highly important.

## 6: Subscribe To My Newsletter To Know When I Publish New Books.

I already mentioned this earlier; I love to connect with my readers. This is just another avenue for me to connect to you. As such, if you would love to know whenever I publish new books and blog posts, subscribe to my newsletter at http://bit.ly/2fantonpubnewbooks. You will be the first to know whenever I have fresh content!

# My Other Books

As I already mentioned, I write books on all manner of topics. In this part of the book, I have categorized them all for easy reading. If you wish to receive notifications about a certain category of books, I have provided a link below every category to ensure you only receive what you are looking for.

## Weight Loss Books

You can search for the titles on Amazon.

## General Weight Loss Books

The books in this category will help you lose weight irrespective of the approach you are using i.e. dieting or workout. I recommend you have them even if you are on specific diets or using specific workouts for weight loss.

**Binge Eating: Binge Eating Disorder Cure: Easy To Follow Tips For Eating Only What Your Body Needs**

**Lose Weight: Lose Weight Fast Naturally: How to Lose Weight Fast Without Having To Become a Gym Rat or Dieting Like a Maniac**

**Lose Weight: Lose Weight Permanently: Effective Strategies on How to Lose Weight Easily and Permanently**

**Get updates when we publish any book about weight loss: http://bit.ly/2fantonweightlossbooks**

## Weight Loss Books On Specific Diets

## Ketogenic Diet Books

KETOGENIC DIET: Keto Diet Made Easy: Beginners Guide on How to Burn Fat Fast With the Keto Diet (Including 100+ Recipes That You Can Prepare Within 20 Minutes)- New Edition

KETOGENIC DIET: Ketogenic Diet Recipes That You Can Prepare Using 7 Ingredients and Less in Less Than 30 Minutes

Ketogenic Diet: With A Sustainable Twist: Lose Weight Rapidly With Ketogenic Diet Recipes You Can Make Within 25 Minutes

Ketogenic Diet: Keto Diet Breakfast Recipes

Get updates when we publish any book on the Ketogenic diet: http://bit.ly/2fantonpubketo

## Intermittent Fasting Books

Intermittent Fasting: A Complete Beginners Guide to Intermittent Fasting For Weight Loss, Increased Energy, and A Healthy Life

Get updates when we publish any book on intermittent fasting: http://bit.ly/2fantonbooksIF

## Any Other Diet

**Get updates when we publish any book on any other diet that will help you to lose weight and keep it off:** http://bit.ly/2fantonsdietbooks

## Relationships Books

Wedding: Budget Wedding: Wedding Planning On The Cheap (Master How To Plan A Dream Wedding On Budget)

How To Get Your Ex Back: Step By Step Formula On How To Get Your Ex Back And Keep Him/her For Good

SEX POSITIONS: Sex: Unleash The Tiger In You Using These 90-Day Sex Positions With Pictures

Money Problems: How To Solve Relationship Money Problems: Save Your Marriage By Learning How To Fix All Your Money Problems And Save Your Relationship

Family Communication: A Simple Powerful Communication Strategy to Transform Your Relationship with Your Kids and Enjoy Being a Parent Again

**Get updates when we publish any book that will help you improve on your personal and professional relationships:** http://bit.ly/2fantonsrelations

## Personal Development

Body Language: Master Body Language: A Practical Guide to Understanding Nonverbal Communication and Improving Your Relationships

Subconscious Mind: Tame, Reprogram & Control Your Subconscious Mind To Transform Your Life

Get updates when we publish any book that will help you become a better person by boosting your productivity, achieving more of your goals, beating procrastination, breaking bad habits, forming new habits, beat stress, building your self-esteem and confidence and much more: http://bit.ly/2fantonpubpersonaldevl

## Personal Finance & Investing Books

Real Estate: Rental Property Investment Guide: How To Buy & Manage Rental Property For Profits

MONEY: Make Money Online: 150+ Real Ways to Make Real Money Online (Plus 50 Bonus Tips to Guarantee Your Success)

Money: How To Make Money Online: Make Money Online In 101 Ways

Get updates when we publish any book that will help you up your game in personal finance and investing: http://bit.ly/2fantonpersfinbooks

## Health & Fitness Books

PMS CURE: Easy To Follow Home Remedies For PMS & PMDD

Testosterone: How to Boost Your Testosterone Levels in 15 Different Ways Naturally

Hair Loss: How to Stop Hair Loss: Actionable Steps to Stop Hair Loss (Hair Loss Cure, Hair Care, Natural Hair Loss Cures)

Hashimoto's: Hashimoto's Cookbook: Eliminate Toxins and Restore Thyroid Health through Diet In 1 Month

**Get updates when we publish any book that will help you up your game in health and fitness: http://bit.ly/2fantonhealthnfit**

## Book Summaries

This category will feature summaries of some of your favorite books, written in a manner you can easily digest and follow:

Summary: The Millionaire Next Door: The Surprising Secrets of America's Wealthy

**Get updates whenever we publish new book summaries:** http://bit.ly/2fantons

## All The Other Niches

This category of books includes anything that we cannot realistically fit in the categories above. As always, if you want just about anything you can get to read, this is the category for you!

### Travel Books

<u>**Kenya: Travel Guide: The Traveler's Guide to Make The Most Out of Your Trip to Kenya (Kenya Tourists Guide)**</u>

### Dog Training

<u>**Dog Tricks: 15 Tricks You Must Teach Your Dog before Anything Else**</u>

### World Issues Books

<u>**ISIS/ISIL: The Rise and Rise of the Islamic State: A Comprehensive Guide on ISIS & ISIL**</u>

**Get notifications when we publish books on anything else above from the niches I mentioned above:** http://bit.ly/2fantonpubnewbooks

# See You On The Other Side!

See, I publish books on just about any topic imaginable!

If you have any suggestions on topics you would want me to cover, feel free to get in touch:

**Website**: http://www.fantonpublishers.com/

**Email:** Support@fantonpublishers.com

**Twitter**: https://twitter.com/FantonPublisher

**My Ketogenic Diet Books Page: https://www.facebook.com/pg/Fast-Keto-Meals-336338180266944**

**Facebook Page**: https://www.facebook.com/Fantonpublisher/

**Private Facebook Group For Readers:** https://www.facebook.com/groups/FantonPublishers/

**Pinterest**: https://www.pinterest.com/fantonpublisher/

PS: You can subscribe to my mailing list to know when I publish new books:

Hey! This is not the entire list! You can check an updated list of all my books on:

**My Author Central**: amazon.com/author/fantonpublishers

**My Website**: http://www.fantonpublishers.com

# Stay With Me On My Journey To Making Passive Income Online

I have to admit; my writing business makes several six figures a year in profits (after paying ourselves salaries). Until recently, I didn't realize just how hard we worked to build this business to what it has become so far.

However, while it is profitable and I want to do it in the long term, I understand its limitations. I know I cannot have an endless number of writers at a time especially if we are to continue delivering high quality products to our customers and readers consistently.

That's why I have recently started getting more serious with self-publishing to help me build a passive income business i.e. income that is not pegged on the number of writers and hours that we put to develop our products.

Thanks to my vast experience and dedication to get things done, I am committed to building a six figure passive income publishing business.

To make sure you are part of this journey, I am inviting you to subscribe to our newsletter (http://bit.ly/2fanton6figprogress) to know my progress as far as passive income generation is concerned. That's not all; if making passive income, just like me, is something you'd love to venture into, you can follow my 'tell it all' blog, which

I explain everything I have done to promote every book and how the results are turning out with figures and images.

My goal is to make sure that while I add value to my audience through the different topics that I publish about to solve various problems for instance, I also add massive value to readers in ways that go beyond just one book. Subscribe to our newsletter to know when I publish new books, how I did market research, how I make money with the books and much, much more.

You can even ask questions on anything you want me to answer regarding publishing and everything else related to the topics of discussion.

**Antony**

**Website**: http://www.fantonpublishers.com/

**Email:** Support@fantonpublishers.com

**Twitter**: https://twitter.com/FantonPublisher

**Facebook                                        Page**:
https://www.facebook.com/Fantonpublisher/

**My        Ketogenic        Diet        Books        Page:**
**https://www.facebook.com/pg/Fast-Keto-Meals-**
**336338180266944**

**Private        Facebook        Group        For        Readers:**
https://www.facebook.com/groups/FantonPublishers/

**Pinterest**: https://www.pinterest.com/fantonpublisher/

I look forward to hearing from you!

# PSS: Let Me Also Help You Save Some Money!

If you are a heavy reader, have you considered subscribing to Kindle Unlimited? You can read this and millions of other books for just $9.99 a month)! You can check it out by searching for Kindle Unlimited on Amazon!

Printed in Great Britain
by Amazon